Glow from the Inside Out

Glow Up Skincare

Minimal Steps. Maximum Glow.
All Skin Tones Welcome.

STEPHANIE WILLIAMS, MBA

BOOKED & BRANDED
PUBLISHING

Copyright

Disclaimer

This book is not medical advice. Always patch test new products and consult a dermatologist for personalized skincare recommendations. Results may vary. Use of this information is at your own risk.

Contents

Introduction   01

Dedication   02

Why Skincare Matters   03

Know Your Skin Type   05

The Glow Up Approach   07

Your Daily Glow Routine (AM/PM)   09

Weekly Treatments & When to Use Them   11

Peptides, Retinols, and Red Light — The Power Players   13

Contents

Weekly Schedule for Glow Goals   15

Lifestyle Habits That Glow Up Your Skin   17

My Morning + Night Routines   19

30-Day Glow Up Tracker   21

Recommended Products (With Cost-Effective Swaps)   23

About The Author   25

Work With Me   27

Glossary/References   28

Introduction

Welcome to Glow Up Skincare, your no-nonsense guide to glowing skin with minimal steps and maximum results. This book is especially for women of color (though everyone is welcome here!), women in their 30s and 40s, and anyone who's tired of routines that cost a fortune and deliver crumbs.

I built this routine during my own glow-up journey—one rooted in simplicity, smart science, and a splash of strategy. I wanted skin that looked vibrant without needing 15 products, expensive lasers, or filters. So, I did what any business-savvy skincare nerd would do—I tested, tweaked, and tracked until I found the glow.

Now I'm handing you the exact system, product list (with prices!), and 30-day tracker that helped me look in the mirror and say, "Okay queen, we see you."

Ready? Let's glow.

Ditch the Drama, Embrace the Glow

Dedication

To My Incredible Readers:

This book is dedicated to you. To every woman who has ever felt overwhelmed, overlooked, or unsure of her path —whether in her skincare journey, her health goals, or her professional aspirations. It's for the queens ready to simplify, strategize, and shine. Your journey inspires me, and it is my deepest hope that these pages empower you to unlock your fullest potential and truly step up your game.

To every woman who has ever looked in the mirror and wished for just a little more glow — this is for you. May your skin radiate confidence, and may you glow unapologetically.

 Where hustle meets strategy.

01

Why Skincare Matters

Skincare isn't vanity. It's self-respect. It's protection. It's a celebration of the skin you live in every single day. A consistent, intentional skincare routine isn't just about looking good — it's about feeling powerful in your own skin. Especially after 35, your skincare habits either support your glow or sabotage it.

02

Know Your Skin Type

Before you build a routine, you need to know what you're working with. The four main skin types are:

Oily: Shiny, especially in the T-zone. Prone to breakouts.
Dry: Tight, dull, sometimes flaky.
Combination: Oily in some areas (like the forehead), dry in others.

Sensitive: Reacts easily to products, weather, or stress.

Pro tip:

Your skin type can shift with seasons, hormones, and age. Pay attention!

03

The Glow Up Approach

We don't do 12-step routines over here. You're busy. You're powerful. You need skincare that works — not just looks cute on the shelf.

Here's our philosophy:

- Minimal steps, maximum results
- Focus on performance, not trends
- Consistency > perfection
- Good skin is built, not bought

**Skincare isn't just about products.
It's about you.**

04

Your Daily Glow Routine (AM/PM)

Let's keep this simple and smart.

Morning Routine (AM):

- Gentle Cleanser (non-stripping)
- Vitamin C Serum (brightening + antioxidant)
- Moisturizer (lightweight or hydrating)
- Sunscreen (broad spectrum SPF 30 or higher — non-negotiable)

Evening Routine (PM):

1. Cleanser (double cleanse if you wear makeup/SPF)
2. Hydrating Serum (like Hyaluronic Acid)
3. Peptides or Repair Serum (optional)
4. Moisturizer (richer at night)

Optional:

Red light therapy 3–5x a week for firmness + glow.

05

Weekly Treatments & When to Use Them

To level up your glow, add these 1–3x per week:

- Clay mask (for oil and pore control) – 1x/week
- Chemical exfoliant (AHA/BHA peels) – 1x/week
- Hydrating mask or overnight mask – as needed
- Spot treatments (if breaking out) – targeted use

Never use a peel and mask on the same day. Alternate and give your skin recovery time.

06

Peptides, Retinols, and Red Light — The Power Players

These aren't your everyday skincare steps. These are your "glow vault" products. The secret weapons. The not-every-day, but oh-so-worth-it when used correctly kind of steps.

Peptides: The Firmness Friend

Peptides are amino acid chains that act like messengers to tell your skin, "Hey, build more collagen!" This means firmer, plumper skin with fewer fine lines. Look for:

- The Ordinary Multi-Peptide + HA Serum (affordable)
- SkinMedica TNS Advanced+ Serum (luxury)

Use peptides on clean skin, ideally at night. Don't mix with exfoliants or strong retinoids in the same routine.

Retinol: The Glow Accelerator

Retinoids are a type of Vitamin A that increase cell turnover. Translation: dull skin peels off, revealing baby-fresh glow beneath. Start slow — 1–2x/week — and moisturize generously.

Look for:

- CeraVe Resurfacing Retinol Serum (drugstore)
- SkinCeuticals Retinol 0.3 or 0.5 (mid-tier)
- Shani Darden Retinol Reform (luxury)

Red Light Therapy (Optional but Powerful)

Try:

- Solawave Red Light Wand
- Dr. Dennis Gross LED Face Mask (splurge-worthy)

Pro Tip:

Only introduce one of these power players at a time, and never after a peel or exfoliant night.

07 Weekly Schedule for Glow Goals

Here's how to build your Glow Week using the products we've covered:

Day	AM Routine	PM Routine
Monday	Cleanse + Vitamin C + SPF	Cleanse + HA serum (optional) + Moisturizer
Tuesday	Cleanse + Vitamin C + SPF	Cleanse + Clay Mask + Moisturizer
Wednesday	Cleanse + Vitamin C + SPF	Cleanse + Moisturizer + Peptides
Thursday	Cleanse + Vitamin C + SPF	Cleanse + Stridex Pad + HA or Moisturizer
Friday	Cleanse + Vitamin C + SPF	Cleanse + Retinol or Peptides + Moisturizer
Saturday	Cleanse + Vitamin C + SPF	Cleanse + Peel + Moisturizer
Sunday	Cleanse + Vitamin C + SPF	Cleanse + Peptides + Red Light Therapy (optional)

Mirror your hand care routine at night too — same actives, same glow!

08

Lifestyle Habits That Glow Up Your Skin

Products can only take you so far. Want to upgrade your entire look? Start here:

- Water: Minimum 75 oz/day — hydration = plumpness.
- Sleep: Aim for 7–8 hours. Skin heals itself overnight.
- Sweat: Exercise gets blood flow going. Bonus: sweat purges pores.
- No alcohol: Go easy here — alcohol dehydrates and inflames.
- Sugar: Sugar stiffens collagen (yes, for real). Cut it back, glow forward.
- Stress: Cortisol shows up on your face. Journaling, breathwork, or walks help.

> *Because skincare isn't just about products. It's about you.*

09 My Morning + Night Routines

Here's what my real-life routine looks like — simple, powerful, consistent.

Morning

1. Gentle Cleanser (La Roche-Posay)
2. Vitamin C (SkinCeuticals C E Ferulic)
3. Moisturizer (CeraVe PM)
4. Sunscreen (Black Girl Sunscreen SPF 30)

Evening (Varies by Day)

1. Cleanser (Osmosis)
2. Active (Stridex, Clay Mask, Peel, Retinol, or Peptides)
3. Hydrator (HA or Peptide serum)
4. Moisturizer (CeraVe PM)
5. Red Light (optional)

> *Minimal Steps. Maximum Glow*

Where hustle meets strategy.

10 30-Day Glow Up Tracker

Track your results daily with the free printable or digital tracker. Check in on:

- Glow (1–10)
- Texture smoothness
- Skin tone evenness
- Firmness and bounce
- Pore visibility
- Under-eye area

Track AM/PM product use and hydration too.

Scan for printable tracker & digital copy.

11

Recommended Products (With Cost-Effective Swaps)

Category	Luxury Product	Cost-Friendly Swap
Vitamin C	SkinCeuticals C E Ferulic ($182)	Maelove Glow Maker ($32)
Cleanser (AM)	La Roche-Posay ($16)	CeraVe Hydrating Cleanser ($13)
Cleanser (PM)	Osmosis Cleanse ($44)	Vanicream Gentle Cleanser ($10)
Moisturizer	Skinfix Barrier+ Cream ($50)	CeraVe PM Lotion ($13)
Retinol	SkinCeuticals Retinol 0.5 ($88	CeraVe Resurfacing Retinol ($22)

Recommended Products
(With Cost-Effective Swaps)

Category	Luxury Product	Cost-Friendly Swap
Peptides	SkinMedica TNS Serum ($295)	The Ordinary Multi-Peptide Serum ($17)
Sunscreen	Supergoop Unseen Sunscreen ($38)	Black Girl Sunscreen SPF 30 ($16)
Clay Mask	Fresh Umbrian Clay Mask ($58)	Aztec Secret Healing Clay ($10)
Peel	Dr. Dennis Gross Peel Pads ($88)	The Ordinary AHA 30% + BHA 2% ($9)
Red Light Device	Dr. Dennis Gross LED Mask ($435)	Solawave Wand ($149)

About The Author

Stephanie Williams, MBA— Strategic Business Consultant, author, and builder of beauty, brains, and business.

Where hustle meets strategy.

Stephanie Williams is a results-driven professional with a passion for helping women glow from the inside out — in skincare, business, and life. With a perfect GPA and an MBA concentrated in Entrepreneurship from the prestigious Jack Welch Management Institute, she brings over a decade of experience in corporate sales, real estate, and brand consulting into everything she creates.

After building multiple six-figure ventures and publishing bestselling digital products, Stephanie launched **Booked & Branded Publishing** — a premium ghostwriting and eBook strategy firm dedicated to helping ambitious professionals turn their expertise into income.

Her own skincare transformation, fueled by science-backed routines, glowing discipline, and late-night Google research (let's be real), inspired this book. Stephanie believes that skincare should be simple, effective, and inclusive — and that confidence is the ultimate glow.

When she's not building empires or testing a new face mask, you'll find her sipping chlorophyll water, walking off stress on a treadmill incline, or helping clients step their game all the way up.

Connect with Stephanie:

✉ **hello@bookedandbrandedpublishing.com**

🌐 **https://www.bookedandbrandedpublishing.com/**

Work With Me

Where hustle meets strategy.

Loved the book? Want a custom routine, a brand collaboration, or help launching your own skincare line or eBook?

Visit: www.bookedandbrandedpublishing.com

Email: hello@bookedandbrandedpublishing.com

Let's build something powerful—together.

Glossary

- AHA/BHA – Exfoliating acids that remove dead skin cells.
- Peptides – Chains of amino acids that signal collagen production.
- Retinol – Vitamin A derivative that speeds up skin renewal.
- HA (Hyaluronic Acid) – Attracts moisture to the skin.
- SPF – Sun Protection Factor. Prevents sun damage and aging.

References

1. American Academy of Dermatology Association – Retinol Benefits and Side Effects
2. Cleveland Clinic – What Peptides Do for Your Skin
3. Harvard Health – Skin Benefits of Vitamin C
4. National Library of Medicine – Red Light Therapy Review
5. Dermstore & Allure Product Archives – Consumer product ratings and reviews

Where hustle meets strategy.

www.ingramcontent.com/pod-product-compliance
Lightning Source LLC
Chambersburg PA
CBHW040132270326
41929CB00005B/35